# No
# Toe Jam

## How To Stop Foot Odor

# No
# Toe Jam

How To Stop Foot Odor


By


Pat Ross

# No
# Toe Jam

Copyright © 2020 by Pat Ross

All Rights Reserved

Printed in the United States of America

Printing History

First Printing:  December, 2020

This is a nonfiction book and all thoughts and views are based on the author's opinion only.

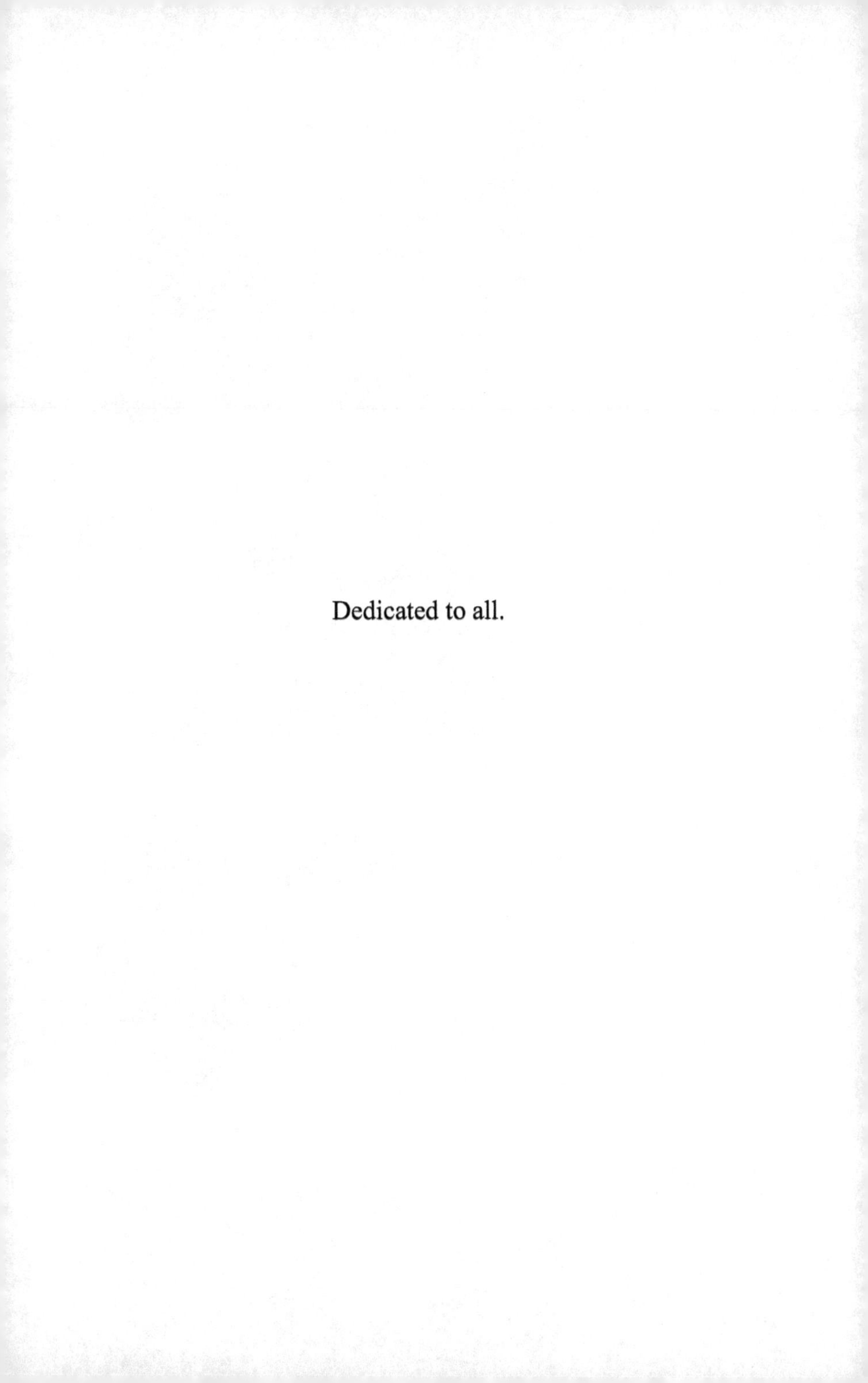

Dedicated to all.

# INTRODUCTION

Frankly, a lot of people do not properly clean their feet when bathing or taking a shower. This can lead to your feet having a bad odor. Most people never learn this simple method I detailed in this book to rid their feet of this foul odor and not spend their entire adult life with those embarrassing funky feet. In this book you will learn how to stop stinky feet forever!

Pat Ross

## No Toe Jam

Truthfully, not all people have smelly feet, but if you do or know someone that does have smelly feet, you will find this book very useful to rid your feet of this odor.

No Toe Jam


Basically, not properly cleaning your feet will most likely lead to a horrible odor.

Pat Ross

No Toe Jam

As a kid I used to have this foot
odor and my entire bedroom
reeked of the funky smell.  The
odor would hit you as soon as
you walked into my room.  Or
whenever I took my shoes off.

Pat Ross

# No Toe Jam

I was so embarrassed by the odor; I did not want anyone in my room and I was reluctant to take my shoes off away from home.

Pat Ross

## No Toe Jam

Seriously, I would wash my feet every day in the shower, but the odor would not go away.

Pat Ross

No Toe Jam

Ironically, my uncle had stinky feet also.  His feet smelled the worst!  The smell was so bad that you could not even enter his bedroom. I then began to think if my toe jam was hereditary.  Until my uncle no longer had smelly fit!

Pat Ross

No Toe Jam




I approached my uncle one day
and told him that I had funky
feet and asked him how did he
get rid of the smell?

Pat Ross

No Toe Jam




What he told me changed my
life forever!

No Toe Jam




He told me, "washing your feet
is not good enough, you have
to     clean between each toe!"

Pat Ross

No Toe Jam




Yes.   Take a lathered soapy
towel and scrub between each
toe!

Pat Ross

No Toe Jam


I ran to take a shower, lathered
my towel, and took my time
scrubbing between each toe.

No Toe Jam

I played basketball the next day
and got in a good sweat to test
my uncle's advice.

Pat Ross

Unbelievable, the funky smell
was gone!

Pat Ross

# No Toe Jam

Toe Jam is caused by bacteria that forms between your toes form not thoroughly cleaning them.

Pat Ross

No Toe Jam




The End